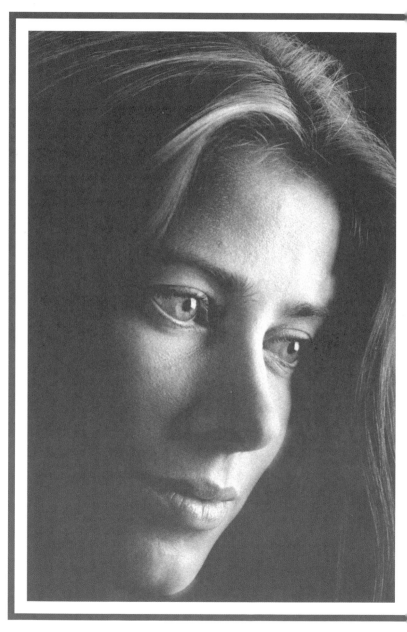

HELP
YOURSELF
to **HEALTH**

Depression

Practical ways to restore health
using complementary medicine

PROF. EDZARD ERNST
MD, PH.D., FRCP (EDIN)

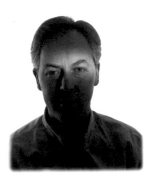

 A GODSFIELD BOOK

Library of Congress Cataloging-in-Publication Data Available

10 9 8 7 6 5 4 3 2 1

Published in 1998 by Sterling Publishing Company, Inc.
387 Park Avenue South, New York, N.Y. 10016

DESIGNED AND EDITED BY
THE BRIDGEWATER BOOK COMPANY LTD

Designer Andrew Milne
Editor Fiona Corbridge
Picture research Lynda Marshall
Illustrations Paul Collicut, Michael Courteney, Ivan Hissey,
and Andrew Milne
Studio Photography Zul Mukhida

Distributed in Canada by Sterling Publishing
c/o Canadian Manda Group, One Atlantic Avenue, Suite 105
Toronto, Ontario, Canada M6K 3E7
Distributed in Australia by Capricorn Link (Australia) Pty Ltd
P.O. Box 6651, Baulkham Hills, Business Centre, NSW 2153, Australia

Printed and bound in Hong Kong

ISBN 0-8069-7066-9

The author would like to acknowledge Dr. Julia Rand's assistance
in writing this book and thank Clare Stevinson for her
thoughtful revision of the manuscript.

CONTENTS

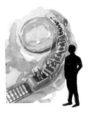

INTRODUCTION

DEPRESSION IS COMMON. *It comes in a confusing array of guises. There are mild forms of depression that can go unnoticed, and there are severe, debilitating forms. Sometimes depression lasts only for a short period, sometimes it comes and goes, and sometimes it is an almost constant, prolonged affliction.*

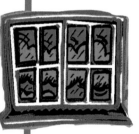

ABOVE *Some days the whole world looks dark, wet, and gloomy.*

Depression affects millions of people worldwide. It results in much distress, suffering and loss of income. Estimates suggest that at least a third of the population will suffer from depression at some point in their lives. Despite its prevalence, there is still a lot of ignorance and misunderstanding about the disorder. Its diagnosis is often missed by busy healthcare professionals. The stigma attached to depression by the public often discourages recognition and treatment.

This book is aimed at people who are affected by depression, both sufferers and those close to them. It will guide you through the maze of complicated issues, inaccessible data, and difficult terminology. We will avoid using scientific jargon

ABOVE *Glimpsing better times ahead is a spur to recovery.*

and the oversimplification of information. Foremost, this book will provide practical help and down-to-earth advice. Depression can be a truly devastating disease – if we can make its burden just a little lighter, we have reached our goal.

Effective conventional treatments exist: medication and cognitive behavior therapy. But what do complementary therapies have to offer? It is important to understand the options, their possibilities and limitations. This book will give you clear guidance, based on the best available research evidence.

LEFT *We all have a darker side to our personality which sometimes overwhelms us.*

WHAT IS DEPRESSION?

Depression is not a new problem – it has been part of the human condition since time immemorial. A variety of names have been used to describe it: melancholy, the vapors, fading away, reclusiveness, or a decline.

HISTORY

As long ago as 1600 B.C., the Ancient Egyptians were using plant remedies to combat melancholia. They also prescribed dancing, listening to music, and sleeping in temples! Late Greek and Roman medicine employed herbal extracts of poppy and mandrake, foods such as barley gruel and asses' milk, as well as gymnastics, massage and baths.

Arabic doctors working in the ninth and tenth centuries used entertainment as well as alcohol, caffeine, opium, and cannabis. In medieval Europe, the approach to mental disorders was less humane and burdened by superstition, with segregation and confinement common. It was only in the second half of the twentieth century that effective new drug and "talking" therapies were developed. Today, there is an increasing willingness to look at other approaches such as herbal medicine, exercise, and massage. It is perhaps rather ironic that we are returning to the methods of the Ancient Greeks.

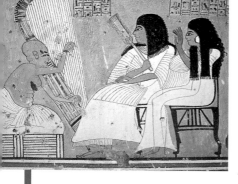

LEFT *Even thousands of years ago, people had depression remedies.*

FAMOUS PATIENTS

Depression affects people from all walks of life. Prominent figures such as Queen Victoria, Abraham Lincoln and Winston Churchill have all been sufferers. Churchill even coined the term "black dog" as a label for his periods of depression. Many individuals from the fields of arts and literature have been sufferers: the composer Robert Schumann, the painter Vincent Van Gogh, the poet Samuel Taylor Coleridge, and the writers Ernest Hemingway and Virginia Woolf. Marilyn Monroe was another famous victim, and the British comedian Spike Milligan has courageously described his sufferings in a book.

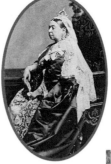

LEFT *Queen Victoria ruled Britain from 1837–1901.*

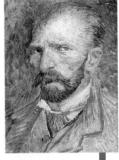

RIGHT *Van Gogh's paintings reflected his intense emotions.*

BELOW *Winston Churchill (1874–1965) was British Prime Minister during World War II.*

RIGHT *Marilyn Monroe's public face concealed private troubles.*

DEPRESSION IS A VERY COMMON PROBLEM

Many people are affected by depression. Figures estimating the scale of the problem vary depending on how depression is defined, and on how closely the population is examined for the symptoms of depression. There is a poor detection rate of the disorder by general physicians. And some sufferers will not seek help, perhaps because they are afraid of the stigma that is still attached to mental illness.

STATISTICS

Depression has been called the common cold of psychiatry because of its frequency. It has been estimated that at any one time, at least 5 percent of the population is suffering from depression. Surveys on depression indicate that at least a third of the population is likely to experience an episode of depression during their lifetime. The scale of individual suffering and of the costs to society in terms of time taken off work and the provision of care which must be funded, is therefore considerable.

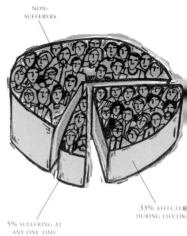

NON-SUFFERERS

33% AFFECTED DURING LIFETIME

5% SUFFERING AT ANY ONE TIME

ABOVE *It's surprising how many people suffer from depression.*

THE EXPERIENCE OF DEPRESSION

Depression is a frightening experience which makes people feel isolated and without hope. Everybody has their own experience of it, and may find it very difficult to express to others, let alone be able to explain these feelings. Although it can be virtually impossible to believe when in the grip of depression, the vast majority of people recover fully.

HOW IS DEPRESSION RECOGNIZED?

To diagnose depression, physicians have developed a method of interviewing and examining patients to detect a constellation of features characteristic of depression.

Sometimes the physician will ask the patient to fill out a questionnaire. The answers provided can be converted to a rating scale to measure the presence and degree of depression.

It is important that physicians actively look for depression. When they visit their physician, people usually do not say they think that they may be depressed. They may present with a minor physical problem, which can throw the physician off the scent.

DEPRESSIVES TALKING

"I looked around me at the other people on the bus. I couldn't understand how the older ones could possibly have got to the age they had, as life was so terrible. Every day was an ordeal."

✧

"My interest in my family and hobbies dried up, I didn't want to do anything, withdrew from people, and couldn't stop crying."

✧

"It seemed as though I was trapped and powerless to change my feelings of gloom and misery. I became frightened and anxious about the future and lost hope of any improvement, so I didn't want to carry on."

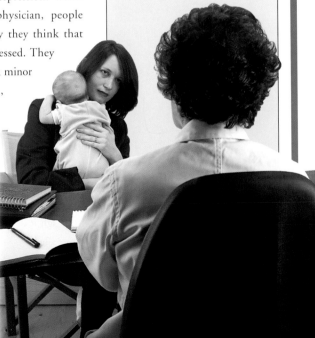

RIGHT *Physicians must ask patients specific questions to diagnose depression.*

HOW DO YOU KNOW IF SOMEONE IS DEPRESSED?

When someone is depressed the main feature is a persistent low mood, or a general loss of interest and enjoyment in things which were previously absorbing or pleasurable. A number of other symptoms can occur as well. For instance, the person may experience difficulty in concentrating, often accompanied by continual feelings of tiredness and a general lack of energy, where even minor tasks become a huge effort.

Sleep patterns may be disturbed: either waking very early in the morning and not being able to get back to sleep, or sleeping for much longer than usual. Loss of appetite and lack of enjoyment of food may occur. The person may feel very pessimistic about the future. Overall self-confidence may be reduced, which makes carrying out the tasks of everyday living even harder. Some people develop deep feelings of guilt, blaming themselves for their difficulties, past actions, and inability to take care of their

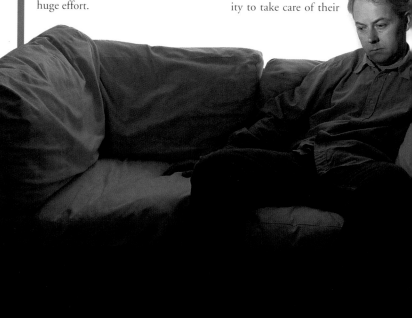

family. In severe cases, they may want to end their life. Each case is different. Even typical symptoms may not be present in some instances (called masked depression). This often renders the diagnosis of depression a difficult task.

A MEDICAL DEFINITION OF DEPRESSION

To diagnose major depression, a physician will look for a certain set of features persisting for at least two weeks (see box), such as not sleeping properly. This is done by observing the patient and talking with him or her. Sometimes further background information is gathered from friends and relatives, who may have noticed changes which not even the depressed person is aware of.

LEFT *Listlessness and lack of interest in life are typical symptoms.*

It is quite common for people who are not clinically depressed to show some of these features, which usually do not persist for a long time. Along with periods of sadness, these are all part of the human experience, and do not represent depression.

DIAGNOSING MAJOR DEPRESSION

For at least two weeks there must be:

☐ Depressed mood and/or loss of interest and enjoyment.

Plus other symptoms from this list making a total of at least five:

☐ Disturbed sleep or excess sleep.

☐ Appetite change, weight loss or gain.

☐ Mental and physical slowing down or agitation.

☐ Poor concentration or indecisiveness.

☐ Tiredness, loss of energy.

☐ Feelings of worthlessness or excessive guilt.

☐ Recurrent thoughts of death or suicide.

TYPES AND MECHANISMS OF DEPRESSION

Psychiatrists now describe and classify depression according to its severity. Some of the older classifications, such as "endogenous" and "reactive" depression are now outdated (but explained in the next section, in case you come across them). Depression is divided into three categories: mild, moderate, or severe.

These categories are based on the number of symptoms present, their severity, and how much the patient concerned is affected by them in everyday life. Mild depression is characterized by the presence of only five or six of the symptoms listed in the box on page 13. It has little impact on the person's ability to function normally. In contrast, in severe depression most of the symptoms listed will be present with greater intensity, and these will have a clear impact. This may show itself as an inability to work or to care for children, and a reduction in usual social activities and the maintenance of relationships with others.

MILD
(5 OR 6 SYMPTOMS)

MODERATE

SEVERE

RIGHT
Depression is classified into three types.

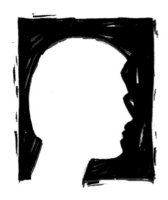

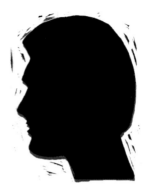

ENDOGENOUS DEPRESSION
*Has no clear cause. High
proportion of vegetative
symptoms.*

REACTIVE DEPRESSION
*Brought on by a stressful event.
Psychological symptoms
predominate.*

ENDOGENOUS AND REACTIVE DEPRESSION

In the past, depression was described as either "endogenous" or "reactive." In cases of endogenous depression, no clear precipitating factors were obvious – the name itself means "arising from within." This type of depression was viewed as the most severe, with the patient suffering from a greater proportion of so-called "somatic" or "vegetative" symptoms.

Reactive depression was thought to be caused by an extreme version of the normal reaction to stress, particularly related to stressful life events such as unemployment, or feelings of loss brought on by the failure of a relationship, divorce, or bereavement. It was believed to be generally milder than the endogenous form, with psychological symptoms predominating.

This division is artificial. Many individuals show features overlapping between the two groups.

MANIA AND BIPOLAR DEPRESSION

A small proportion of people with depression will also experience mania. When this happens, the problem is then known as bipolar disorder. This name is used because two extremes or poles on the scale of mood occur: both high mood (mania) and low mood (depression). Consequently, depression alone is sometimes termed unipolar disorder. When mood is abnormally and persistently high, the term mania is used. In some cases, the person becomes irritable rather than euphoric.

During a manic phase, people may think themselves capable of anything and embark on risky business ventures, sexual relationships, and spending sprees. They may believe that they have a special relationship with a public figure, or that they have produced revolutionary inventions. Speech is often very rapid, allowing no interruptions and jumping rapidly from one subject to another. The need for sleep may be reduced, energy seems boundless, libido and appetite are increased, and socially inappropriate behavior may occur. The person concerned is usually unaware that there is a problem.

Mania tends to come on rapidly, particularly after stressful events. Untreated, it may last for weeks or months, but generally has a shorter duration than episodes of depression, and is likely to end more abruptly. Various orthodox drug treatments may be prescribed for the control and prevention of mania.

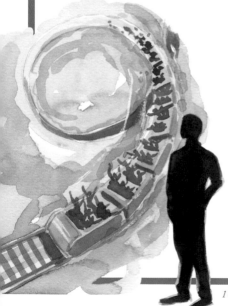

BELOW *The extreme "high" of mania causes loss of normal perception.*

POST-NATAL DEPRESSION

This expression describes depression in a mother, in the weeks or months following childbirth. About half of new mothers experience a mild brief mood reduction, often known as the "baby blues." In around 5 to 20 percent of all new mothers, a depressed mood develops. It is severe in a small minority of cases (about 1 in 500), and then it is vital that professional help is sought. The mother may experience depressive feelings of guilt, inability to cope, and hopelessness related to her new role.

The causes of post-natal depression are complex and involve a number of different factors. During pregnancy there is a huge increase in sex hormones, such as oestrogen and progesterone. Once the baby is born, hormone levels drop abruptly. This could be one cause. However, it is by no means certain that the hormone changes alone produce the depression, as not all women get depressed and the evidence is largely circumstantial. There are all sorts of social and psychological factors at play after a birth, when new responsibilities and demands are present. For instance there may be money or relationship difficulties, or a perceived lack of emotional or practical support.

POSSIBLE CAUSES OF
POST-NATAL DEPRESSION

◇ *Hormonal changes*
◇ *Lack of sleep*
◇ *New, inescapable responsibilities*
◇ *Change in role from wage-earner to dependant*
◇ *Change in relationship with partner*
◇ *Lack of support*

LEFT *Up to 20 percent of new mothers experience depression.*

SEASONAL AFFECTIVE DISORDER

Seasonal affective disorder (aptly abbreviated to SAD) is a condition where depressed mood occurs in a regular cycle at a particular time of the year, usually the winter, with mood improving in the spring and summer.

SAD tends to be characterized by increased sleeping, overeating, lethargy, and despair.

Generally, it is believed that the lowering of mood results from biochemical changes produced by reduced light levels in the winter. One theory is that the decrease in light causes a small gland at the base of the brain, called the pineal gland, to produce more melatonin. Melatonin production takes place during the hours of darkness and helps to make people drowsy. In animals, melatonin plays a part in reducing activity and increasing sleep during the winter. When bright light hits the eye it has the effect of stopping the production of melatonin. Consequently, bright light is thought to help those who appear to have SAD, and various appliances are commercially available which will administer light during the hours of darkness.

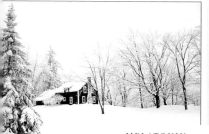

January

	TUE	WED	THUR	FRI
			1	2
	6	7	8	9
	13	14	15	16
	20	21	22	23
	27	28	29	30

MELATONIN

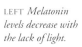

LEFT *Melatonin levels decrease with the lack of light.*

WHAT CAUSES DEPRESSION?

Depression is likely to involve a complex mix of biological, social, and psychological factors. Some personal characteristics may make an individual more likely to develop the disorder, and certain stressful factors coming from outside may act to trigger off depression.

Scientific investigations indicate that actual changes in brain chemistry occur during depression, but it is not clear how or why these changes start. This knowledge has stimulated the discovery of new drugs, which work by helping to restore the balance of brain chemistry.

BELOW *Personality is shaped by a mix of factors.*

DO PHYSICAL DISEASES CAUSE DEPRESSION?

Diseases directly affecting the brain may produce depression. Examples include people who have had a stroke, Parkinson's disease, multiple sclerosis, or a head injury. Some infectious diseases such as influenza, glandular fever, or viral hepatitis are often followed by depression. Unusual glandular diseases such as an underactive thyroid, or insufficient cortisol production, can result in depression. Even some prescribed drugs may cause depression as an unwanted side-effect. One example of this is the oral contraceptive pill, which in rare cases can cause depression. Depression can also be a feature of the use of illicit drugs such as cocaine and amphetamines, or of chronic excess consumption of alcohol.

DOES DEPRESSION RUN IN FAMILIES?

There is some evidence that close relatives (parents, children, brothers and sisters) of an individual who suffers from severe depression have a somewhat increased chance of developing depression themselves. For the milder forms of depression, no link has been detected. In the majority of cases of depression, there is no apparent familial connection. This indicates that, generally speaking, the genetic instructions inherited from our parents do not have a very strong direct link to the likelihood of developing depression. For a few people, their genes may make them more vulnerable to the disorder, but this is not necessarily the case even if other family members have been affected. One reason for this is that a large number of factors are involved in the development of depression. Studies of identical twins show that even if two individuals have identical genetic make-up and one develops depression, it does not necessarily mean that the other will suffer from the same disorder. No specific gene for depression or a clear pattern of inheritance have been discovered.

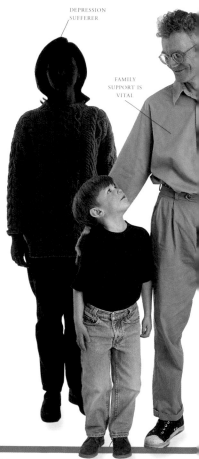

DEPRESSION
SUFFERER

FAMILY
SUPPORT IS
VITAL

RIGHT *Mild
depression is not
usually inherited
by children.*

CHARACTERISTICS OF DEPRESSION

✧ Thoughts tend to be gloomy, negative and intrusive.

✧ Feeling a failure at relationships or life in general.

✧ Feelings of guilt.

✧ Thinking illogically and drawing general conclusions from single events.

PSYCHOLOGICAL FACTORS AND DEPRESSION

If a friend does not greet you in the street, you would normally assume that it is because he did not see you. But if you are depressed, you might assume it is because he does not like you, and become preoccupied with negative thoughts about the event.

In this way a vicious circle may become established so that mood spirals downwards, and it can then be difficult to break out of it. It is not clear which comes first, the depression, or the negative way of thinking. Whichever it is, negative thinking is a part of depression. It sustains it and probably even deepens it.

This knowledge has been put to good purpose in the "talking" treatment known as cognitive behavior therapy, which has been proved to be effective (see page 35).

ABOVE
Negative thinking reinforces depression, preventing recovery.

CHILDREN NEED TO HAVE THE ILLNESS EXPLAINED TO THEM

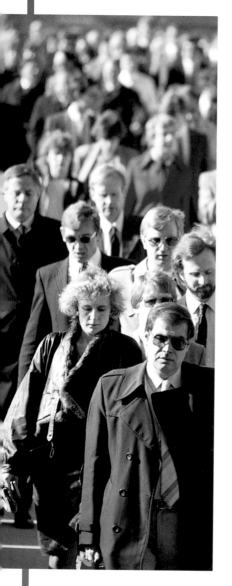

STRESS AND DEPRESSION

The risk of developing depression is increased in the weeks or months after stressful life events such as bereavement, job loss, or financial difficulties. (However, for many people suffering depression, there will be no obvious event linked to the way they feel.) It seems that these major events can act as a trigger for initiating depression.

Sometimes the trigger is an accumulation of events, or the effect of a long-term situation such as marital discord. Loss – either material or emotional – may be followed by depression. Other life events including marriage, moving, or retirement may be involved. Isolation, particularly in elderly people living alone, can increase vulnerability to depression. Features such as the lack of a confiding relationship, or a history of having been abused as a child, can make a person more vulnerable to depression when stressful events take place.

LEFT *The build-up of everyday stresses can lead to depression.*

BRAIN BIOCHEMISTRY
AND DEPRESSION

The communication system in the brain consists of a complex interconnecting network of millions of elongated nerve cells. Electrical impulses travel along these, and have to be carried over a minute gap between each cell, called a synapse. Chemical messengers, called neurotransmitters, carry the signal across. The levels of certain chemical neurotransmitters are reduced in depression. Although it is not yet understood just how or why these messengers become unbalanced, the development of antidepressant drugs has revolutionized the treatment of depression.

A number of different neurotransmitters exist. The main types involved with depression are thought to be norepinephrine (noradrenaline in the UK) and serotonin. The brain is an incredibly complex organ and its functioning is not fully understood. Yet our current level of knowledge does allow us to use various drug treatments to significantly relieve the symptoms of depression.

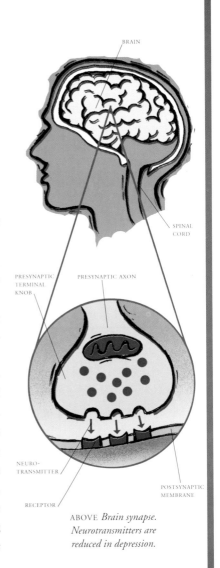

BRAIN

SPINAL CORD

PRESYNAPTIC TERMINAL KNOB

PRESYNAPTIC AXON

NEURO-TRANSMITTER

RECEPTOR

POSTSYNAPTIC MEMBRANE

ABOVE *Brain synapse.*
Neurotransmitters are
reduced in depression.

CONVENTIONAL DRUG TREATMENTS FOR DEPRESSION

Although many psychological and social factors are at play in the development of depression, there are also biochemical changes taking place in the body, particularly in the brain. Antidepressant drugs act to restore these biochemical changes to normal, and lift depression in the majority of people.

DO ANTIDEPRESSANT DRUGS WORK?

As with any drug, antidepressants may produce some unwanted side-effects along with beneficial effects, and so their use has to be carefully supervised by a medical practitioner. Many people feel reluctant to take drugs for an illness such as depression, but their value can be appreciated once it is understood how they work, that they are not addictive, how long they take to work, and their likely side-effects.

Antidepressants may be used as only one part of a treatment plan, along with other therapies.

ANTIDEPRESSANT DRUGS

There are three main groups of antidepressant drugs which act in different ways and have different possible side-effects.

✧ Tricyclic antidepressants
✧ Selective serotonin reuptake inhibitors (SSRIs)
✧ Monoamine oxidase inhibitors (MAOIs)

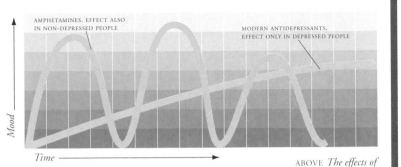

AMPHETAMINES. EFFECT ALSO
IN NON-DEPRESSED PEOPLE

MODERN ANTIDEPRESSANTS.
EFFECT ONLY IN DEPRESSED PEOPLE

Mood

Time

ABOVE *The effects of
mood-altering drugs.*

ANTIDEPRESSANTS ARE NOT ADDICTIVE

Many people are confused about whether antidepressants and tranquilizers are addictive. Tranquilizers such as diazepam have developed a bad reputation because of dependence. Some people become tolerant to them, so that they have to take more and more to have the same effect. When it comes to stopping tranquilizers, unpleasant withdrawal symptoms may occur within a day or two, such as shaking, aches and pains, and feeling hot or cold.

Real antidepressants are not addictive and do not cause these types of problem. Before the discovery of the first antidepressants in the late 1950s and 1960s, stimulants (amphetamines or "pep pills") were the only drugs available for the treatment of depression. Amphetamines can rapidly lift mood, but are soon followed by a severe drop in mood (a "downer"). They are still sought after by illicit drug users.

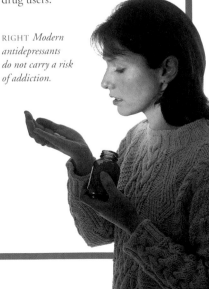

RIGHT *Modern
antidepressants
do not carry a risk
of addiction.*

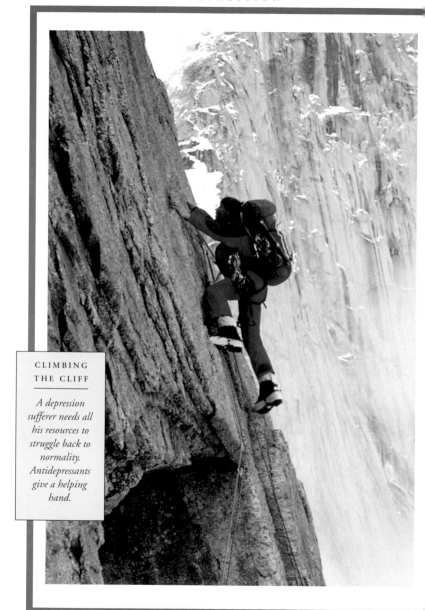

CLIMBING THE CLIFF

A depression sufferer needs all his resources to struggle back to normality. Antidepressants give a helping hand.

In contrast, antidepressants are not in demand by drug users as they are not stimulants, and raise mood only in those with depression, and only after a period of weeks. Thus antidepressants do not possess the major characteristics of addictive drugs: they do not produce immediate pleasure; their withdrawal does not cause an unpleasant reaction needing a further dose of the drug to relieve it. Nevertheless, it is wise not to suddenly stop taking antidepressants without advice. This could increase the risk of the depression returning. The usual practice is to tail the dose off over a month or so.

ANTIDEPRESSANTS TAKE TIME TO WORK

Improvement begins around two to four weeks after starting to take the medication. The rub is that unwanted side-effects are felt rapidly after starting the treatment, and before any improvement is noticeable. Therefore it is important not to give up taking the antidepressants too soon. Various antidepressants each have possible side-effects to be aware of, so that they are not mistaken for a new manifestation of the depression.

The vast majority of the side-effects are not serious, but they can put people off from continuing with the medication. There are many ways around this problem. Usually, when starting antidepressants, the dose is gradually increased so the body gets used to the drug. Side-effects also commonly disappear with time, as the body adapts. If the side-effects are very troublesome, it is possible to change to another medication.

It is recommended that antidepressants are taken for at least six months after recovery, and sometimes for two years. This greatly reduces the chance of depression occurring again.

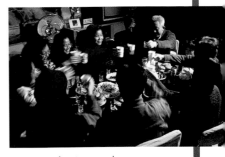

ABOVE *Medication must be continued for a time after recovery.*

TRICYCLIC ANTIDEPRESSANTS

The tricyclic antidepressant drugs are named after the three rings in their chemical structure. They act by increasing the availability in the brain of the chemical messengers (neurotransmitters) norepinephrine and serotonin. Imipramine was the first tricyclic antidepressant to be discovered, in the 1950s. Many other types of antidepressant have since been developed from the drug imipramine. They all seem to be similarly effective in treating depression, but differ in their side-effects.

SIDE-EFFECTS OF TRICYCLIC ANTIDEPRESSANTS

Unfortunately tricyclic antidepressants do not just act on neurotransmitters involved with depression. They also affect other systems causing unwanted effects, such as dry mouth, constipation, tremor, blurred vision, urinary retention and a drop in blood-pressure when getting up, making falls a risk. Other possible side-effects are sleepiness, weight gain and, more rarely, irregularities in the rhythm of the heart or an increased risk of epileptic fits. Not everyone will experience these side-effects to any degree.

DRUG TYPES

There are several different tricyclic antidepressants. As well as the scientific or "generic" name there is often one or more trade names applied to the same substance – amitriptyline (Tryptizol®), imipramine (Tofranil®), and dothiepin (Prothiaden®).

BELOW *Tricyclic drugs have a three-ringed chemical structure.*

THE CHEMICAL STRUCTURE OF DIBENZAZEPINE DRUGS, PARENT OF IMIPRAMINE

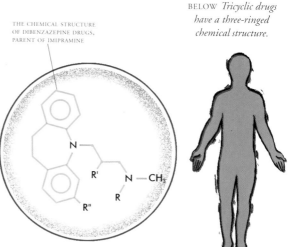

SELECTIVE SEROTONIN REUPTAKE INHIBITORS (SSRIs)

The SSRI group of antidepressant drugs has been introduced recently and has received much publicity and hype. Attention has focused especially on fluoxetine (Prozac®). The other main members of the group are fluvoxamine (Faverin®), paroxetine (Seroxat®), and sertraline (Lustral®). The SSRIs specifically act to increase serotonin levels at synapses between brain cells, by reducing the level of its reuptake. This results in more serotonin being available for nerve impulse transmission in the brain.

Unlike the tricyclic antidepressants, the effect is mainly on serotonin rather than also on norepinephrine or other neurotransmitters such as acetylcholine. SSRIs work as well as tricyclics in depression, but there is less information available on their long-term safety.

SIDE-EFFECTS OF SSRIs

SSRIs have fewer side-effects than the tricyclics, but may produce nausea with or without vomiting, and insomnia. For some people the general lack of a sedating effect is an advantage, but for others with anxiety and sleeplessness it is not. Other side-effects include dizziness, headache, tremor, diarrhea and restlessness. SSRIs are less likely than tricyclics to cause weight gain or disturbances to the rhythm of the heart.

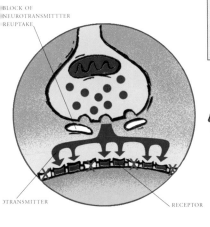

BLOCK OF
NEUROTRANSMITTTER
REUPTAKE

OTRANSMITTER

RECEPTOR

LEFT *SSRIs reduce serotonin neurotransmitter reuptake.*

MONOAMINE OXIDASE INHIBITORS (MAOIs)

MAOIs are not as commonly used as the other classes of antidepressant, largely because they can have serious side-effects and interact with various foods and drugs. They can be useful for treating depression with less common features, such as phobias. They are thought to work by inhibiting the enzyme (monoamine oxidase) which is responsible for breaking down monoamines within cells. The neurotransmitters serotonin and norepinephrine are examples of monoamines. The result is that enough neurotransmitter is then available to restore mood and lift depression.

MAOIs take three to five weeks or sometimes longer to work. Phenelzine (Nardil®), isocarboxazid (Marplan®) and tranylcypromine (Parnate®) are examples of MAOIs.

More recently, other drugs have been developed, which are termed reversible inhibitors of monoamine oxidase type A (RIMA for short). RIMAs such as moclobemide (Manerix®) are safer to use, as there is less chance of adverse interactions with other substances.

BELOW *Monoamine pathways in the brain and spinal cord.*

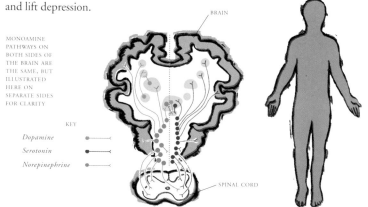

MONOAMINE PATHWAYS ON BOTH SIDES OF THE BRAIN ARE THE SAME, BUT ILLUSTRATED HERE ON SEPARATE SIDES FOR CLARITY

KEY

Dopamine

Serotonin

Norepinephrine

BRAIN

SPINAL CORD

SIDE-EFFECTS OF MAOIs

MAOIs inhibit the enzymes which normally break down a range of substances known as monoamines. This increases the monoamine neurotransmitters, norepinephrine and serotonin, which are believed to be responsible for the improvement in depression. However, at the same time, other amines such as tyramine and dopamine are no longer broken down properly. If someone taking MAOIs eats foods containing tyramine, there is a sudden and dangerous increase in blood pressure. Foods which need to be avoided include cheese, pickled herring, broad bean pods, some wines, and yeast extracts.

The enzyme inhibition can last for two weeks after the drug has been stopped.

MAOIs also interact with many other drugs including some over-the-counter cold remedies. This means that great care has to be taken to avoid problems. Patients are normally issued with a warning card summarizing this information. Other effects are similar to those caused by tricyclic antidepressants, for instance dry mouth, dizziness and constipation.

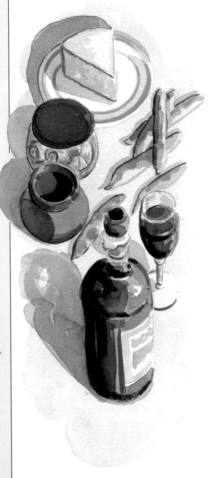

BELOW *Certain foods must be avoided when taking MAOIs.*

NON-DRUG TREATMENTS FOR DEPRESSION

In psychological approaches to the treatment of depression, discussion between the patient and a therapist is used to help the problem. These methods are sometimes termed "talking treatments." General supportive advice, information, and explanation should be available from medical staff to all patients with depression.

Psychological approaches tend to be popular as they do not involve pills, and provide time and attention from a therapist. This gives the patient reassurance that the problem is being taken seriously.

The problem with the more specialized forms of psychological approach is that where they are available, the demand usually outstrips the supply so that long waiting lists can develop. As these therapies are time-consuming, they are also expensive, which in turn affects their availability.

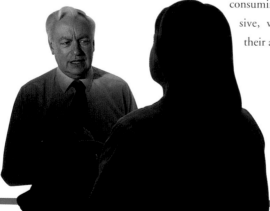

LEFT *Counseling can be of great help in restoring a balanced approach.*

PROBLEM SOLVING

1 *Examine your life for sources of worry and tension.*

2 *Focus on the problem areas.*

3 *Look at methods of attacking the problems.*

4 *Follow a strategy for self-help.*

5 *Review your achievements and the success of chosen strategies.*

COUNSELING

In many respects, counseling is an extension and refinement of everyday ways of helping distressed people. It takes place on a one-to-one basis between a therapist and a client. There are many forms, using different approaches and emphases. A counselor can create a professional relationship which helps to sustain the patient. Listening helps the patient to feel understood and reassured. As well as providing information and advice about depression, the counselor can encourage the expression of emotion and the sharing of feelings, which can help to make the patient feel better. The counselor can help to improve morale by agreeing achievable goals with the patient and encouraging self-help. Problems may be reviewed, and in some forms of counseling step-by-step problem-solving strategies are taught and implemented.

It is important that care is taken to find a well-qualified, reliable counselor (see chapter on "Choosing a Complementary Therapist"). While in the vulnerable state of depression, the danger of becoming over-dependent on a therapist should be recognized.

PSYCHODYNAMIC PSYCHOTHERAPY

This type of psychological therapy may take place over years, rather than weeks or months. Sessions generally last about fifty minutes, once or twice a week. There is a greater emphasis on the dynamics of the relationship between the therapist and the patient. The aim is to enable the sufferer to recognize the unconscious factors believed to relate to the disorder, so gaining understanding and control over feelings and actions.

Its techniques are derived from psychoanalysis and are based on key analytical concepts. For instance, Freud's ideas of psychosexual development may be used to try to gain an insight into subconscious motives arising as the individual grows up, which may affect later life. Not everyone accepts Freud's views, so the value of the approach is controversial. Free mental association is used as the main method of recall, as this is thought to throw up significant memories which can then be interpreted. The interpretation of dreams (where images are believed to be loaded with significance, often of a sexual nature) is seen to be important.

There is no clear evidence that psychodynamic psychotherapy speeds the process of recovery, and in some instances focusing on past events may encourage introspection and guilt. The general view is that psychodynamic psychotherapy is of limited value in depression, and is anyway only possible in less severe cases where attention and memory are not impaired.

RIGHT *Psychodynamic therapy examines past life events of the patient.*

COGNITIVE BEHAVIOR THERAPY

What is cognitive behavior therapy? This rather unwieldy term describes a method designed to change patterns of thinking and behavior which interfere with the natural processes of recovery from depression. Rather than investigating the causes of depression, the therapy focuses on teaching people how to control their disturbed thoughts, emotions and behavior, which act to maintain, and perhaps even deepen, low mood. The patient works closely with a therapist, often a clinical psychologist.

Interestingly, cognitive behavior therapy has been shown to be as effective as drugs in mild to moderate forms of depression. However, drugs tend to be used more frequently as they are less time-consuming and cheaper. Cognitive behavior therapy usually consists of between six and twenty hour-long sessions, taking place at weekly intervals.

Although it has not been established whether negative thought patterns precede the development of depression, or if they simply develop during it, three main types of disordered thinking in depression have been identified. Ways of tackling these are discussed on the next pages.

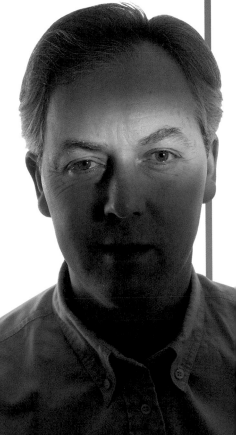

BELOW *Patients learn to focus on their thought processes.*

CHALLENGING NEGATIVE THOUGHTS

It is common for depressed people to experience gloomy, intrusive thoughts, which the mind keeps returning to. These negative thoughts seem to reinforce and deepen the depressed mood. In cognitive behavior therapy, the patient is asked to keep a diary to record feelings, thoughts and events throughout each day. These are later discussed with the therapist, and the patient learns how to challenge the negative thoughts. For example, if a patient believes that only bad things happen to him or her, by looking at the past it would be possible to discover positive experiences and happy times and events. Or perhaps the patient believes herself to be worthless, and unacceptable to other people. The therapist will guide the patient into looking for evidence which contradicts this belief. Raising awareness like this helps the patient to break out of the cycle of thinking negatively, and to start to generate feelings of hope for the future. The patient learns how to recognize and challenge negative thoughts as they occur, and with time this can help to reduce their frequency and break the downward spiral of mood.

BELOW *Keeping a diary of your thoughts is helpful.*

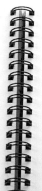

MONDAY
Dog ran off. PANIC!
What if he gets run over?

TUESDAY
Row with David. We can't seem to get on with each other these days. Feel very LONELY.

WEDNESDAY
Dog reappears. Make a big fuss of him. We both have chocolate drops. Feel a bit better.

FRIDAY
Went out with David for a meal. Managed to discuss my feelings without being aggressive. Maybe there's some hope for us!!

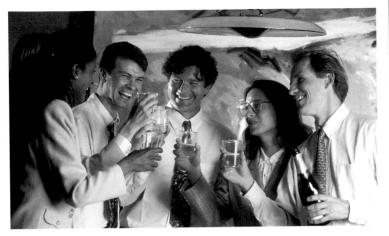

ABOVE *Learning to accept yourself will allow you to be relaxed in company.*

CHALLENGING UNREALISTIC EXPECTATIONS

Some depressed people hold unrealistic expectations about the world so that when things do not turn out as they think they should, it undermines their confidence and happiness. They may, for instance, believe that they cannot be happy unless they are liked by everyone, and that they should never get angry with people. By discussing this belief, it becomes clear that it would be an impossible task to be liked by everyone, and that people are able to achieve happiness without this happening.

Once the distorted way of thinking is recognized, patients may conclude that making more effort to meet and get to know new people, without the pressure of believing that it is essential that everyone likes them, would free them to enjoy friendships again. Therapists encourage patients to identify their own unrealistic beliefs, consider how these affect their lives, and work out how to change things for the better.

CHALLENGING ILLOGICAL WAYS OF THINKING

It is not uncommon for depressed people to think in illogical ways which tend to maintain the depression, such as drawing a negative general conclusion from one small incident. For instance, they may believe that because a friend did not telephone, the friend no longer wants to know them. A therapist would help the depressed person to conclude that this one incident could be explained in a number of other ways (such as the friend being very busy), and other evidence could be uncovered to show that there was an ongoing friendship between the two people.

It is easy to look at the black side of things when depressed. Cognitive behavior therapy aims to help patients to become aware of unhelpful thought patterns and behavior, so that they can take control and make progress on the road to recovery.

CHALLENGING INACTIVITY

Inactivity and social withdrawal are common features of depression. As patients gradually go out less and often withdraw from life, they receive less stimulation and have fewer opportunities for positive experiences. One way to help to get the ball rolling again is to develop a written task plan.

LEFT *Life is a matter of perspective: is this glass half empty or half full?*

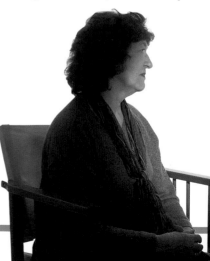

RIGHT *Cognitive behavior therapists gently expose thought patterns.*

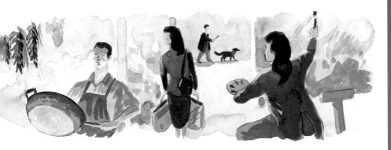

ABOVE *Plan a spread of activities during the day.*

For example, the job of cleaning the house may seem completely overwhelming. By breaking it up into individual components, and tackling the simplest chores first, it will then seem much more manageable. It is important not to set unrealistic goals. When a task is completed, this helps to develop a sense of achievement and control which gradually helps to lift mood and to prevent a downward spiral.

Activity scheduling is another helpful approach. Patients keep a record of what they do during each hour, and are encouraged to rate their sense of accomplishment or pleasure after each activity. This can then be used to help to decide which activities to increase in frequency because they produce feelings of mastery and pleasure, or alternatively which produce problems to be tackled. Scheduling activities increases the chance of patients doing them, and greater activity in turn helps to improve mood. Sometimes distraction is a useful technique: getting involved in an absorbing activity occupies the mind and helps to block out unwelcome unpleasant feelings and thoughts, which may attempt to intrude.

ELECTROCONVULSIVE THERAPY (ECT)

Electroconvulsive therapy, also called electroshock therapy, is a specialized hospital-based therapy which is now only used in very severe cases of depression where life is in danger, or when all other approaches have failed. It suffers from a bad reputation as a barbarous method, as depicted for instance in the film *One Flew Over The Cuckoo's Nest*. Yet it can be a safe and effective treatment when used for certain specific categories of patient. The principle of ECT is that the induction of a fit can relieve depression. This was discovered accidentally in the 1930s in Italy, during the search for a treatment for schizophrenia.

Today, ECT consists of giving the patient a short-acting anesthetic plus a drug to relax the muscles, and then applying an electric current for a split second to the brain to induce a fit. Electrodes are placed on the temples, and the electric shock causes the patient to lose consciousness during the convulsion. The ECT is given once or twice a week, with a course

ECT
✧ Can be effective in well-defined cases.
✧ Has probably been over-used in the past.
✧ Requires a specialized setting.
✧ Is not free of side-effects.

of treatment lasting for perhaps six to eight treatments. It produces a rapid improvement in the majority of patients. So far it is not understood exactly how ECT works, just that it has a beneficial effect. Serious complications due to the treatment are rare. However, it may produce short-term impairment of memory in some people.

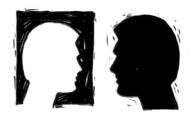

ABOVE *ECT was an offshoot of schizophrenia treatment research.*

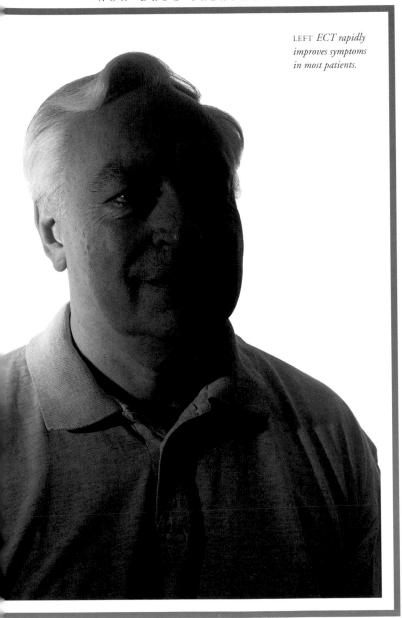

LEFT *ECT rapidly improves symptoms in most patients.*

COMPLEMENTARY THERAPIES

The terms "complementary" or "alternative" therapies cover a wide variety of approaches and techniques, some more respectable than others. This diversity can present a confusing and puzzling picture to anyone trying to find a therapy for their particular health problem.

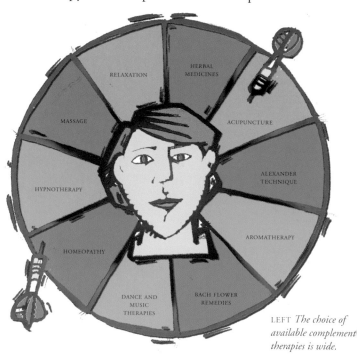

RELAXATION

HERBAL MEDICINES

MASSAGE

ACUPUNCTURE

HYPNOTHERAPY

ALEXANDER TECHNIQUE

HOMEOPATHY

AROMATHERAPY

DANCE AND MUSIC THERAPIES

BACH FLOWER REMEDIES

LEFT *The choice of available complement*
therapies is wide.

We aim to provide a guide through this maze – to describe what has scientifically been shown to work in depression, and to suggest what holds promise, while outlining the pitfalls and uncertainties. Armed with this information, you can make informed decisions about your way forward.

LEFT *Check out the therapies before you decide which to try.*

People in Western nations have been turning to complementary therapies in increasing numbers. Surveys in different countries have shown that 25–75 percent of the population have tried complementary therapies in the last year. Reasons for this growing popularity include a disillusionment with orthodox medical approaches, failure to find relief with conventional medicine for chronic long-term conditions, a growing willingness to try new methods, the need for time and attention from a caring therapist, and a desire for treatments which are seen to be more "natural" and therefore thought to be free from unwanted side-effects.

SIDE-EFFECTS

"Natural" products and methods are not necessarily free of risks. This is a common misconception.

HOW DO YOU FIND OUT WHAT WORKS?

Depression is one of the commoner disorders for which people turn to complementary medicine for a solution. So how do you decide where to start when faced with the perplexing array of choices? If you look at general books on complementary medicine, particularly those written by practitioners, all sorts of therapies are proposed as a treatment for depression.

How is it possible to find out if any of these really work, or if they involve unexpected hazards? The scientific way is to carry out an extensive search for published evidence among scientific literature, and this has been done by us at Exeter University, UK. While anecdotal stories about individuals who have improved after a particular treatment can be revealing, firmer evidence is still needed.

In clinical medicine, the most reliable method for establishing whether or not a treatment works is known as the randomized controlled trial. This rather off-putting term describes a fairly simple idea. Two or more groups of people who are comparable at the start of the study (achieved by random

BELOW *Randomized controlled trials test a treatment against a placebo.*

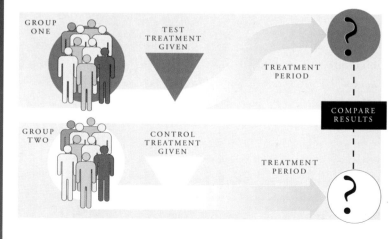

GROUP ONE

TEST TREATMENT GIVEN

TREATMENT PERIOD

COMPARE RESULTS

GROUP TWO

CONTROL TREATMENT GIVEN

TREATMENT PERIOD

allocation) are compared after receiving the treatment under investigation (the experimental group), or another intervention (the control group). Sometimes the experimental group will be compared with a group receiving an existing treatment which has already been shown to work, and sometimes it will remain untreated, or receive a placebo or sham therapy. In this way, it is possible to tease out whether the treatment under investigation works better than the one given to the control group.

> **COMPLEMENTARY THERAPIES SHOWN TO WORK BY SCIENTIFIC EVIDENCE**
>
> *Acupuncture*
> ✧
> *Aromatherapy*
> ✧
> *Massage*
> ✧
> *Music therapy*
> ✧
> *Relaxation*

WHICH COMPLEMENTARY THERAPIES HELP IN DEPRESSION?

The amount of research carried out on complementary therapies in the treatment of depression is so far fairly limited. This means that the jury is still out for a lot of therapies, and more good-quality research needs to be funded in this area. However, the good news is that a considerable body of evidence does exist for the benefits in mild to moderate depression of both the herbal remedy St. John's wort (*Hypericum perforatum*), and of physical exercise. Although the amount of evidence for certain therapies is limited, acupuncture, aromatherapy, massage, music therapy and relaxation techniques may be of some value. Anxiety is often a strong component of depression, and many of these therapies are calming.

Where evidence is not yet available regarding the efficacy and safety of a therapy, assess the situation as fully as possible before embarking on a treatment. Always ensure that your health problems have been investigated and properly diagnosed by an orthodox physician before starting a course of complementary therapy.

ST. JOHN'S WORT

Plants are vital for our existence: without them we would not have enough oxygen to breathe or food to eat. Since prehistoric times, plants have provided medicines. Each culture has its own tradition of herbal medicine, handed down verbally or in written herbals and other records.

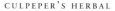

CULPEPER'S HERBAL

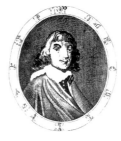

Nicholas Culpeper (1616-1654) published a book called the **Complete Herbal.** *It was a comprehensive guide to self-treatment by herbal medicine. It contained descriptions of medicinal plants, and suggested where they could be found. It also gave instructions on how to prepare remedies from the plants. The book is still available today.*

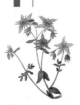

Today, Western medicine largely relies on synthetic drugs. However, it should not be forgotten that many valuable drugs were originally derived from plants, and that undoubtedly many useful plant-based compounds still await discovery.

Among the more well-known branches of herbal medicine are Traditional Chinese Medicine, Indian Ayurvedic medicine, and Western herbalism. They have different theoretical or philosophical backgrounds, but all share the use of plant materials as remedies. Often the underlying philosophy is a holistic approach to treatment which views the body as an integrated whole.

LEFT *Herbal treatments have been around for a long time.*

Lavender (Lavandula augustifolia) combines well with rosemary, kola, and skullcap for treating depression. Gently strengthens the nervous system and encourages restful sleep.

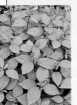

Skullcap (Scutellaria laterifolia) is a nervine tonic and can be used to treat all types of depression. It combines well with valerian.

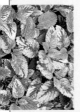

Balm (Melissa officinalis) is a gentle sedative which soothes away stress. It fights digestive problems brought on by depression.

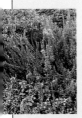

Rosemary (Rosemarinus officinalis) relaxes nervous tension which may give rise to headache, indigestion, or general malaise.

WHAT IS HERBAL MEDICINE?

It is common for herbalists to prescribe mixtures containing plant extracts from many different plant species. As each individual extract can contain many active chemical substances, it is often not known which chemical, or chemicals, are responsible for any beneficial effects. Scientists rarely understand exactly how an extract acts on the body to produce the desired effects on the individual (but it must be established without doubt that the extract reduces symptoms without doing any harm to the patient).

Indeed, the ways in which some synthetic chemical drugs work are not fully understood, but they do have to pass stringent safety tests, and they certainly have to be shown to work clinically. As with any therapy, the balance between wanted effects and adverse reactions has to be carefully weighed up – whenever the potential harm of a treatment outweighs the potential benefit, it is then regarded as obsolete.

HERBAL MEDICINES AND SAFETY

Plants are quite capable of producing toxic substances. The fact that plants occur naturally does not mean that they are necessarily safe. Some of the most deadly poisons known to the human race are plant products. An example is ricin from the castor oil plant, notoriously used on the point of an umbrella to kill the Bulgarian defector, Georgi Markov, in London in 1978. It has even been suggested that the only difference between a safe drug and a poison is

ABOVE *Georgi Markov was killed with ricin poison.*

the dose. This statement applies equally to plant medicines and synthetic drugs. Thus it is crucial that safety studies are carried out. Even if a plant has a long history of use, it is possible that it may have side-effects which are slow to develop or not very obvious, and have been overlooked in the past.

Another safety issue is the mis-identification of the plant species, or the intentional or accidental adulteration of the remedy with toxic materials, or even conventional drugs. The active content is likely to vary according to the source of the plant, the parts of the plant used, and the extraction procedure. Thus it is important that adequate quality control takes place so that the required dose of the correct species is received.

PROBLEMS OF PLANT MEDICINES

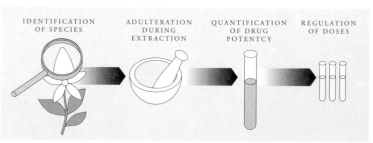

| IDENTIFICATION OF SPECIES | ADULTERATION DURING EXTRACTION | QUANTIFICATION OF DRUG POTENTCY | REGULATION OF DOSES |

TRADITIONAL USES FOR ST. JOHN'S WORT

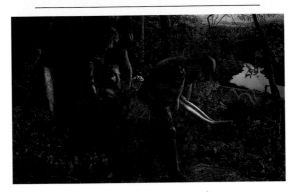

ABOVE *St. John's wort was used to treat wounds sustained in battle.*

St. John's wort has a number of colloquial names including "touch-and-heal," "balm of the warrior's wound," and "sunshine of the soul." It has an ancient history of use as a healing herb, which was recorded as early as the first century by Pliny and Dioscorides. Disorders which it has been used to treat range from wounds, burns and chest infections, to nervous conditions and menopausal and premenstrual problems. This broad diversity of traditional medicinal uses reflects the high number of active chemicals which it contains.

St. John's wort was an important part of the folklore of the Middle Ages because of its healing power and the belief that it could cast out demons. The plant is thought to have become associated with St. John because it flowers around the time of the saint's day in June, and contains a red juice which has been seen as a symbol of the martyred saint's blood.

RIGHT *John the Baptist, the namesake of St. John's wort.*

BOTANICAL CHARACTERISTICS OF ST. JOHN'S WORT

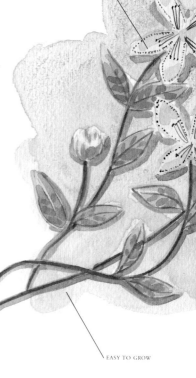

FLOWERS IN JUNE

The variety of St. John's wort used is *Hypericum perforatum*. When the leaves are held up to the light, they appear to have numerous small perforations, hence the name of "perforatum." In fact these are clusters of translucent oil glands. A few other members of this plant family have these glands, but a unique feature of *Hypericum perforatum* is the two raised ridges running down the sides of the stem.

OIL GLANDS

ABOVE *Both leaves and stem contain oil-producing glands.*

EASY TO GROW

ABOVE *The stem, leaves and flowers are used to make the remedy.*

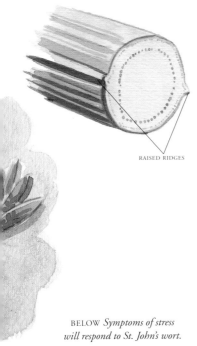

RAISED RIDGES

ST. JOHN'S WORT FOR DEPRESSION

Since the 1980s, European scientific trials have investigated the use of extracts of St. John's wort for treating mild to moderate depression. In 1996, the results of 23 of the most rigorous type of scientific studies (randomized controlled trials) involving 1,757 people, were summarized in the *British Medical Journal.* The overall conclusion of the research was that extracts of St. John's wort are effective in relieving the symptoms of mild and moderate types of depression.

BELOW *Symptoms of stress will respond to St. John's wort.*

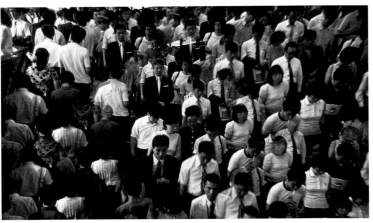

HOW DOES ST. JOHN'S WORT WORK?

Herbal extracts from St. John's wort contain many different chemicals with exotic names such as bio-flavonoids, anthroquinones, diter-penoids, hypericin and pseudo-hypericin. It is not yet clear which of the constituents are responsible for the improvement in the symptoms of depression. Hypericin is thought to be an important component, and good quality extracts are generally stan-dardized to contain a specified amount of this substance. It is crucial that extracts are standardized, and the quality rigorously controlled, so that people can be sure of the dose taken.

The mode of action of St. John's wort has not yet been firmly estab-lished. It is possible that it may act by modulating the serotonin neurotrans-mitter system (see page 23 for an explanation of neurotransmitters), and it may also act on the monoamine oxidase enzymes. Clearly, more work needs to be done before we can be sure just which of the components of the plant are the important ones,

PRODUCING THE REMEDY

St. John's wort contains hypericin, which is thought to be its most valuable ingredient for the treatment of depression.

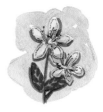

HARVEST
The entire plant growing above the ground is picked – flowers, shoots and leaves.

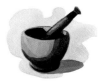

PROCESSING
Plants are processed to extract the valuable constituents.

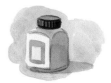

MARKETING
The herbal extracts are made into medicines: pills, capsules, oils, and liquids.

and how they act. It is quite possible that more than one component and mechanism are important, and that a number of interactions take place.

THE SAFETY OF ST. JOHN'S WORT

With any medical intervention, it is likely that as well as beneficial effects, there will be unwanted side-effects. Conventional synthetic antidepressant drugs can produce a range of unpleasant side-effects. St. John's wort has fewer and generally milder side-effects.

The commonest unwanted effects reported with St. John's wort are nausea, stomach ache, skin rashes, itching and tiredness. These problems tend to be mild and to occur in only about 2–3 percent of people. There is a theoretical risk of a skin reaction known as photosensitivity, where the skin becomes sensitized to sunlight. Yet this is highly unlikely to occur at the doses used to treat depression.

RIGHT The sun can be hazardous to people using St. John's wort, as the skin may become sensitized to sunlight.

It seems to be a reversible problem that will disappear if the herbal extract is stopped. Thus St. John's wort is not only an effective antidepressant, but it is also the safest such drug known today. While in Germany it is marketed as a fully licensed drug – where it is the most popular antidepressant of all (including Prozac®) – it is available in the UK and the US as a food supplement and other products.

St. John's wort is a pain-reliever and a sedative, helpful in treating neuralgia and anxiety. When applied externally, its anti-inflammatory effect makes it valuable for rheumatism and sciatica. It will also help to heal sunburn, wounds, and bruises.

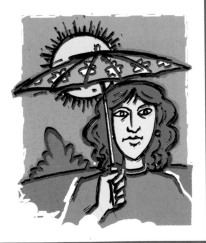

EXERCISE

In the past, most people's lives involved a great deal of physical activity at work or at home. Today, widespread mechanization and the availability of labor-saving devices such as washing machines, lawnmowers, and vacuum cleaners, means that many people are far less active than was common in previous centuries.

The majority of recent scientific studies looking at the effect of exercise on depression, have shown that it is linked to an improvement of symptoms in those suffering from mild to moderate depression. Much of this work has been carried out in the United States. Overall, the link seems to be a strong one. As well as helping people to feel better, exercise has many other health benefits: it reduces heart disease, high blood pressure, strokes, and obesity. It also fights the weakening of bones in osteoporosis.

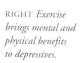

RIGHT *Exercise brings mental and physical benefits to depressives.*

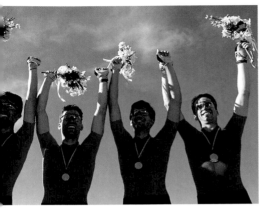

LEFT *A sense of achievement and boosted self-esteem result.*

HOW MIGHT EXERCISE HELP?

It has been suggested that exercise might act in a variety of different ways to improve mood during depression. There are a number of possible psychological explanations for its benefits. For example, exercise can provide a depressed person with a distraction from intruding unhappy thoughts which might otherwise worsen mood. Exercise can result in a sense of achievement, and raise self-esteem and confidence. Another advantage is that it can reduce the feelings of isolation often encountered in depression, by providing opportunities for meeting and chatting to people.

On the physiological level, exercise can improve the fitness and efficiency of the heart and lungs, and help to reduce the symptoms of tension and anxiety which often accompany depression. Exercise may even stimulate the production by the body of chemicals called endorphins, which relieve pain and raise mood. Another possibility is that exercise restores the balance of chemical neurotransmitters such as serotonin and norepinephrine, so that the depression lifts.

It may well be that exercise acts via several of these routes to improve well-being. Other scientific research work has implied that exercise might help to prevent the recurrence of depression. When done correctly, exercise is also very safe and only carries a few health risks. Therefore exercise is well worth considering as part of a strategy for coping with depression.

WHAT SORT OF EXERCISE AND HOW MUCH?

Many types of exercise have been found to be related to improvements in depression. These include activities ranging from walking, dancing, running, cycling, swimming and skipping, to weight training, karate and team sports such as soccer and hockey. Some of these activities are termed "aerobic" exercise. This means that they involve physical work sustained over relatively long periods which improves the efficiency of the heart and lungs, as for example in jogging or swimming. Some "anerobic" exercise, on the other hand, may involve high-intensity work for very short periods, as in weightlifting or sprinting. The good news is that either form of exercise helps depression,

> **MODERATE EXERCISE**
>
> *Good way to start*
> ✧
> *Swimming*
> ✧
> *Walking*
> ✧
> *Stretching exercises*
> ✧
> *Tai Chi or Yoga*
> ✧
> *Cycling*

BELOW *Aerobic exercise sustains a raised pulse rate for a long period.*

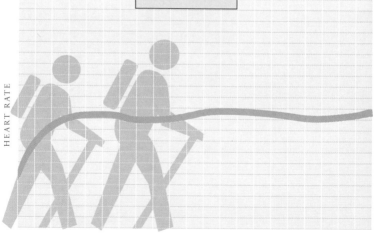

HEART RATE

TIME IN MINUTES

although aerobic exercise is more likely to produce other types of health benefits and therefore is normally preferable. So far no one particular type of exercise has been shown to be superior, so people can select whatever sport they find the most enjoyable.

Beneficial effects have been observed even with exercise of low intensity, where it is not necessary to become physically fit. This is very encouraging, as it means that a strenuous intensive program (which would also be burdened with some risks) is not necessary. Taking exercise three to four times a week is normally adequate to gain benefits. There does not appear to be any advantage (regarding mood) in increasing the frequency beyond this. If sessions last for about thirty minutes, it will be enough to produce an improvement.

> INTENSIVE EXERCISE
>
> ---
>
> *For the fit*
> ✧
> *Tennis*
> ✧
> *Soccer*
> ✧
> *Squash*
> ✧
> *Aerobics*
> ✧
> *Athletics*

BELOW *In anerobic exercise, the pulse rate is very rapid at times.*

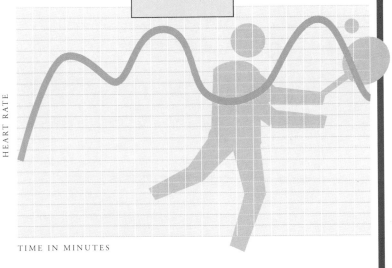

HEART RATE

TIME IN MINUTES

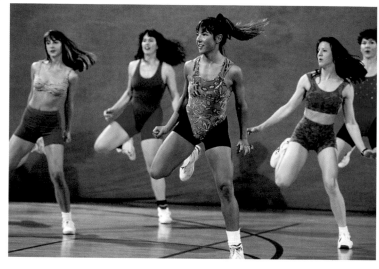

ABOVE *Group exercise sessions help with motivation.*

GETTING STARTED

Exercise provides a wide range of health benefits, so it is very worthwhile. Whatever exercise you choose, remember – it should be fun! While there are all sorts of solo activities, it can help motivation to join a class or group – which also provides company. For people who prefer solo activities, those which do not cost much in terms of equipment include walking, jogging, and swimming.

If you suffer from a chronic health problem such as arthritis or heart disease, it is mandatory to discuss your exercise plans with your physician to make sure that it is safe for you. Inviting a friend or relative to join you in taking up a new activity can help motivation and make it more fun. It is important not to set unrealistic targets or to try to do too much. The best approach is to start off gently, and gradually build up to a level which is comfortable and enjoyable.

Even a little exercise is better than none. Selecting something which you enjoy means that you are more likely to continue with it. Start your program by going for a gentle walk each day. Investigate the availability of local classes in a sport which appeals to you. For some people variety is important: they can have fun trying different types of exercise.

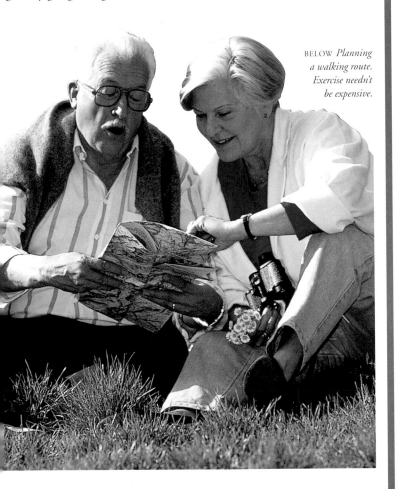

BELOW *Planning a walking route. Exercise needn't be expensive.*

ACUPUNCTURE

Acupuncture is an ancient Chinese form of healing,
involving the stimulation of selected points on the body.
These points are stimulated by inserting fine needles,
or by applying pressure, heat or electricity.
The heat is produced by burning a herb on top
of the needle. This is known as moxabustion.

BELOW *Three important
Chinese physicians.*

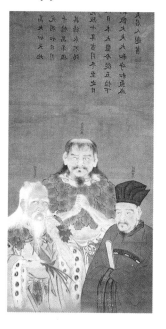

Folklore has it that acupuncture was discovered when Chinese physicians tending wounded soldiers noticed that certain arrow wounds cured chronic disorders or old injuries. By noting where the wounds were, and then experimenting with flint flakes and fishbones, the art of acupuncture was gradually developed. The first textbook, called *The Yellow Emperor's Classic Of Internal Medicine*, was produced some time between 300 and 100 B.C. Acupuncture is just one component of Traditional Chinese Medicine, which also involves herbal medicine, massage, manipulation, relaxation techniques, and attention to the diet.

THE WEST

Acupuncture was unknown in the West until the seventeenth century, when French Jesuit missionaries described it. It was then given the name we know it by, derived from the Latin words for needle (*acus*) and puncture (*punctura*). For a while it became the vogue in France, but then lapsed into obscurity. It came to prominence in the West again in the 1930s, following the publication of a series of detailed works about it by the French diplomat Soulier de Morant. During the 1970s, dramatic television coverage showing Chinese patients having surgery and using acupuncture to control their pain, brought the technique into the public eye in the West and started scientific research into this area.

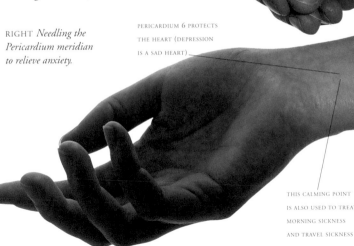

RIGHT *Needling the Pericardium meridian to relieve anxiety.*

PERICARDIUM 6 PROTECTS THE HEART (DEPRESSION IS A SAD HEART)

THIS CALMING POINT IS ALSO USED TO TREAT MORNING SICKNESS AND TRAVEL SICKNESS

ARM TAI YIN

Lung

LEG TAI YIN

Spleen

ARM SHAO YIN

Heart

LEG SHAO YIN

Kidney

ARM JUE YIN

Pericardium

LEG JUE YIN

Liver

ARM YANG MING

Large Intestine

LEG YANG MING

Stomach

ARM TAI YANG

Small Intestine

LEG TAI YANG

Bladder

ARM SHAO YANG

San Jiao

LEG SHAO YANG

Gall Bladder

Bladder

San Jiao

Pericardium

Large Intestine

Lung

Heart

Small Intestine

Stomach

Kidney

Spleen

Liver

Gall Bladder

LEFT *The twelve main meridian channels in the body*

PHILOSOPHY

Traditional Chinese Medicine incorporates complex ancient Taoist philosophy. Put simply, it is believed that energy known as Qi (pronounced "chee") moves in everything, and that it polarizes into the complementary forces of Yin and Yang. These forces are in dynamic balance in a healthy person, producing a state of harmony (Tao). Yin is seen as passive, dark and female, and Yang as the contrary – active, light, and male.

Qi is thought to flow along invisible pathways in the body, called meridians. Ill-health is seen to be a consequence of an imbalance between Yin and Yang, so that the flow of Qi is disturbed. The aim of Traditional Chinese Medicine is to restore the balance of Yin and Yang so that the smooth flow of Qi is regained, which then allows the body to heal itself. Acupuncture is one way of achieving this state of energy balance, by stimulating points on the meridians to unblock energy if it has become stuck, or to speed it up or slow it down.

Twelve paired main meridians are described, which correspond to each of the five Yin and six Yang organs and to the pericardium around the heart. There are believed to be up to 500 acupoints along the meridians. The concept of five elements (wood, fire, earth, metal and water) is also used. These elements are thought to be linked to the organs of the body: wood (Liver and Gall Bladder), fire (Heart and Small Intestine), earth (Spleen and Stomach), metal (Lungs and Large Intestine), water (Kidney and Bladder). Each of the elements must be in harmony for good health.

TREATMENT VIA THE MERIDIANS

Points on the meridians are treated to act directly on their associated organ. The meridians also "communicate" with each other and their related organs, so problems in one area may also be treated via a different channel. As well as the twelve regular channels, there are eight extraordinary channels which are not directly linked to organs. Two of these, the Du Mai and the Ren Mai, have acupuncture points on them.

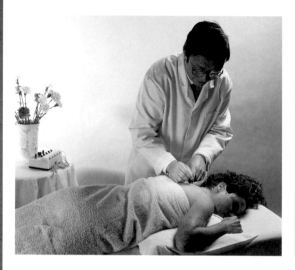

LEFT *Acupuncture may act on the nervous system to treat depression.*

WESTERN ACUPUNCTURE

Acupuncture is also practiced in a modified form known as Western or scientific acupuncture. Many of those practicing scientific acupuncture qualified in orthodox medicine and then went on to receive further training in acupuncture. These practitioners do not adhere to the traditional Chinese explanations as to why or how acupuncture works. Instead, they believe that there are biological mechanisms to explain its effectiveness. Although these mechanisms have not been fully established, it is thought that acupuncture acts by influencing the nervous system.

At local level, acupuncture seems to help to diffuse small areas of irritability (trigger points) remaining in muscles after injury. These trigger points have often been found to correspond to acupuncture points. In addition, acupuncture may well stimulate the release of chemical messengers called neurotransmitters which block pain at the level of the spinal cord. It is possible that acupuncture also affects neurotransmitter levels in the brain. This could be how it helps to treat depression.

DOES IT HELP?

In China, several scientific trials have been carried out on depressed patients to compare the use of acupuncture, or electroacupuncture, with tricyclic antidepressant drugs. (In electroacupuncture, a small electric current is used to stimulate the acupuncture points.) The work showed that acupuncture, and particularly electroacupuncture, resulted in an improvement similar to that produced by the tricyclic antidepressants.

These results are promising, but the research is still in its early stages and so far only involves a small number of patients. The research has been produced mainly by one group of investigators. Essentially the jury is still out as to whether acupuncture helps in depression, although there are indications that it may do. One theory put forward to describe how it may work is that acupuncture could stimulate the amount of the chemical messengers serotonin and norepinephrine in the brain. An imbalance of these chemicals is thought to occur in cases of depression.

WHAT SHOULD I DO IF I WANT TO TRY IT?

Firstly, it is best to discuss this option with your physician. Acupuncture is not totally risk-free: bruising, fainting, and local skin infections can occur, and much more rarely serious complications such as puncturing a lung with a needle (pneumothorax). Needling should be avoided in people with a bleeding disorder or who are taking anticoagulants such as warfarin. Those with a cardiac pacemaker should not have electroacupuncture as this could interfere with the pacemaker. Good practitioners will use disposable needles, or sterilize their needles properly, to avoid the risk of transmitting infections such as hepatitis and HIV.

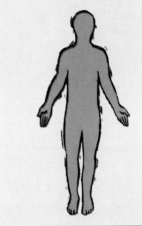

OTHER COMPLEMENTARY THERAPIES

Several other forms of complementary treatment are being advocated for depression. On the following pages, we will briefly explain the most important of these and outline what is known regarding their safety and effectiveness for treating depression.

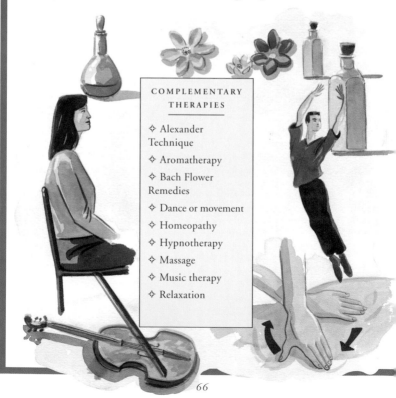

COMPLEMENTARY
THERAPIES

✧ Alexander
Technique
✧ Aromatherapy
✧ Bach Flower
Remedies
✧ Dance or movement
✧ Homeopathy
✧ Hypnotherapy
✧ Massage
✧ Music therapy
✧ Relaxation

ALEXANDER TECHNIQUE

The Alexander Technique aims to correct faulty posture and body movement, which are thought to result in physical and mental tension, put stress on bones, joints and muscles, and to produce poor circulation and shallow breathing. Practitioners are known as teachers, and they help their clients to correct faulty posture and movements. They claim that the technique produces postural harmony, improves circulation and breathing, and creates freedom of movement and relaxation.

The technique was developed by an Australian actor, Frederick Alexander (1869–1955). Alexander had difficulties with his voice on stage, and by observing his own body in mirrors while rehearsing, concluded that poor posture and movement had produced this problem. He then went on to develop a complete system of posture and movement based on achieving a balanced relationship between the positions of the head, neck and the spine.

LEFT *The body is trained into good postural habits.*

EFFECTIVENESS

Alexander teachers claim that the technique can help depression. This claim has not been put to the test in scientific studies: evidence so far is anecdotal.

SIDE-EFFECTS

The technique is a gentle one and is unlikely to cause any adverse effects, provided that the teacher is properly qualified.

TREATMENT

Tuition is usually on a one-to-one basis, and about twenty sessions or more will be

In aromatherapy, essential oils extracted from the flowers, fruit, seeds, leaves and roots of plants are used for healing. The aromatherapist selects the oils according to the physical and emotional state of the client. Oils may be blended together, and are generally massaged (immersed in a carrier oil) into the skin. They may also be inhaled, used in the bath, or applied as a compress. It is thought that each oil has specific effects, for example that lavender oil is calming and neroli improves your mood.

BELOW *Essential oils with different therapeutic properties are used.*

Little scientific work has been carried out to objectively assess the effects of aromatherapy, and it is not known whether it is the essential oils, or the massage, or both, which are responsible for any changes. Many people who have tried aromatherapy believe that it is relaxing, reduces anxiety, and generally helps them to feel better.

Essential oils are powerful mixtures of plant chemicals. They are on unrestricted sale in the UK and the US, often without any instructions on use or safety warnings. They should not be applied directly to the skin in pure form. They can sometimes produce skin reactions, particularly in those with sensitive skins. It is important to be aware that some oils, such as orange, lemon or bergamot, can sensitize the skin to sunlight so that burning can occur much more easily. As the skin absorbs the chemicals from the oils, they are best avoided in pregnancy.

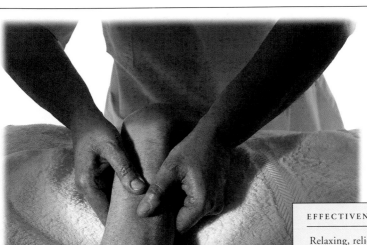

ABOVE *A regular massage is a pleasant addition to other therapies.*

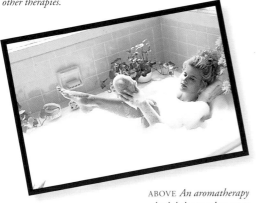

ABOVE *An aromatherapy bath helps to relax away the day's tensions.*

EFFECTIVENESS

Relaxing, relieves anxiety and stress, and helps to improve well-being.

SIDE-EFFECTS

Do not apply essential oils neat to the skin. Avoid certain oils in pregnancy. Some oils sensitize the skin to sunlight. May produce skin reaction.

TREATMENT

An aromatherapy massage lasts about an hour.

BACH FLOWER REMEDIES

Bach Flower Remedies consist of tinctures extracted from flowers. They are prepared by placing petals in spring water in the sun for a few hours, which is then made into a tincture using brandy as a preservative. Remedies are taken by placing drops on the tongue, or drinking them mixed with water. Advocates of the therapy believe that a negative emotional state is the underlying cause of an illness. They claim that flower remedies lift the emotions, and as a result the body is then free to heal itself.

The therapy was developed by Edward Bach, a Welsh homeopathic physician, in the early part of the twentieth century. After experimenting on himself with dew collected from flowers encountered on his country walks, he developed a set of thirty-eight remedies. He recommended particular flower tinctures for specific emotional problems, for instance pine, elm or willow for despair.

REMEDIES

Cherry plum, for the fear of losing control.

Gorse, for hopelessness.

Sweet chestnut, for desolation.

EFFECTIVENESS

There is no scientific evidence to back up the claims for flower remedies, although there are plenty of testimonials of supposed beneficial effects. It is possible that these may be due to placebo effects, for example resulting from the expectation that the tinctures would help.

SIDE-EFFECTS

Safe for people of all ages, with no known side-effects.

TREATMENT

A few drops of flower essence are dissolved in a glass of water, and this is sipped slowly.

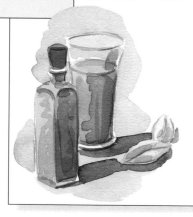

LEFT *Drops of the remedy may be taken with water.*

DANCE/MOVEMENT THERAPY

In dance therapy, movement aims to assist physical and mental healing, and enhance the emotional and physical integration of the individual. It is believed that the opportunity to move freely provides the chance to express feelings and release tension; also that the body and mind are inseparable, so that movements reflect inner emotional states.

Although dance has been part of the human experience for thousands of years, it has only been used as a therapy since the beginning of this century. Dance therapists believe that it has a spectrum of beneficial effects, ranging from improving physical co-ordination, to psychological aspects such as promoting body image, improving self-confidence, and encouraging self-expression.

RIGHT *Poise and confidence are an added bonus.*

They believe that dance helps to unify mind, spirit and body, resulting in a sense of completeness and well-being. As a group activity, it provides opportunities to socialize, and so helps to reduce ingrained feelings of isolation.

EFFECTIVENESS

The amount of good-quality scientific evidence on the benefits of dance therapy in depression is as yet very limited. Only a few studies have been carried out, involving small numbers of patients over short periods of time. There is some indication that dance may help to improve mood, but more work is necessary.

SIDE-EFFECTS

None.

TREATMENT

Dance can be enjoyed at any time.

HOMEOPATHY

Homeopathy was developed by the German doctor Samuel Hahnemann in the late eighteenth century. It is based on the principle of "like cures like" – it is proposed that if a particular substance causes symptoms in a healthy person, it can then be used in very small quantities to cure a disease which produces the same symptoms in a sick person.

To make a remedy, a concentrated solution of a substance is diluted many times. Opponents to homeopathy argue that these much diluted solutions are unlikely to contain even one molecule of the original substance, so they cannot possibly work. Although advocates of homeopathy cannot explain how the solutions might work, it has been suggested that somehow the water molecules preserve a "memory" of the substance, which is effective. The remedies are derived from plant, mineral, or animal materials.

Homeopaths aim to treat the whole person rather than just a symptom, and believe that their remedies stimulate the natural healing processes of the body.

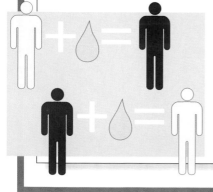

LEFT *The homeopathic principle is "like cures like."*

BELOW Aconitum napellus, *a remedy source.*

EFFECTIVENES

Little scientific work has been carried out on homeopathy for the treatment of depression, although some studies have indicated that it helps in certain other disorders.

SIDE-EFFECTS

Keep your physician informed about treatments.

TREATMENT

Pills, powders, liquids, or ointment.

HYPNOTHERAPY

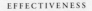

Hypnosis produces an altered state of consciousness in which the subject becomes deeply relaxed, and is influenced by a set of suggestions. The person remains conscious and is aware of what is being said and what is going on around him. Hypnotherapists assert that people cannot be made to do things against their will when they are hypnotized.

Most people can be hypnotized if they want to be. Clients are guided into a hypnotized state by the use of relaxation methods, imagery and visualization techniques.

The therapist may make suggestions aimed at changing the way the client usually experiences or responds to something. Hypnotherapists believe that they can produce rapid results by directly influencing the unconscious mind of their subject, while he or she is totally relaxed.

EFFECTIVENESS

So far there is no scientific evidence that hypnosis can cure depression, and if there are any apparent benefits, they are likely to be short-lived.

SIDE-EFFECTS

Sometimes hypnosis uncovers painful memories, and may even create unpleasant false memories.

TREATMENT

The client is put into a state of complete relaxation, in which he or she remains aware of what is going on.

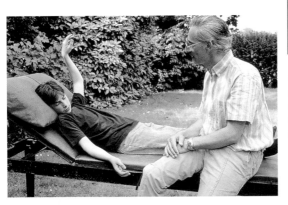

LEFT *Hypnosis subjects become deeply relaxed and open to suggestion.*

MASSAGE THERAPY

Massage consists of a range of manipulative techniques on the muscles and soft tissues of the body. The therapist employs a variety of kneading, rubbing, pressing, and stretching movements. These help to improve blood flow, relax muscles and generally produce a feeling of well-being. The intensity of the massage can vary from soft and gentle stroking to vigorous and uncomfortable pummeling.

MASSAGE AROUND THE WORLD

Swedish or Western massage was developed in the nineteenth century and focuses on toning the muscles.

✧

Oriental massage tends to focus on body points for releasing vitality and promoting mental and physical harmony.

✧

Thai massage aims to clear energy blockages in "energy channels" (meridians).

✧

Japanese reiki therapy uses touch to restore energy.

✧

Tuina is an intense form of deep massage employed as part of Traditional Chinese Medicine.

✧

In India, Ayurvedic marma massage is a very brisk technique used to stimulate specific points on the body.

BELOW *Massage relaxes muscles knotted with tension.*

AN ANTI-STRESS SELF-MASSAGE

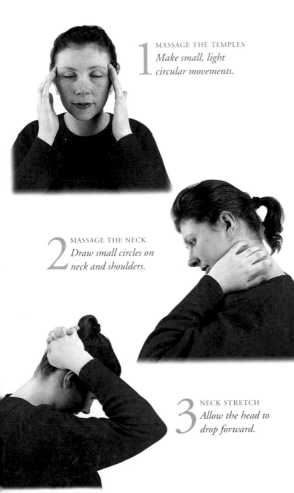

1 MASSAGE THE TEMPLES
Make small, light circular movements.

2 MASSAGE THE NECK
Draw small circles on neck and shoulders.

3 NECK STRETCH
Allow the head to drop forward.

EFFECTIVENESS

Several scientific studies have looked at the effect of massage on depression. The results of trials on Swedish massage suggest that it may help to alleviate the symptoms of depression. This may partly be due to its relaxing effect.

SIDE-EFFECTS

As the treatment is almost entirely free of risks, it can be recommended as an adjunct to antidepressive treatment.

TREATMENT

As frequently as desired, according to finances.

MUSIC THERAPY

Music therapy is based on the belief that we all have an inborn ability to respond to music. Music appears to be able to change mood and arouse emotions.

There are several forms of music therapy: it may involve listening to music, singing or playing music as an individual or in a group setting. The music therapist assesses the patient and then selects appropriate music for the condition, often with a great deal of input from the patient. Music may help to provide a distraction from the current circumstances and aid the recall of pleasant associations from the past.

Many reports about the benefits of music therapy are anecdotal, but there are a few interesting results from the small number of scientific investigations which have been carried out. Most of the studies do not involve the treatment of depression. For instance, premature babies have been shown to put on more weight in intensive care units where music is played. Research shows that music reduces anxiety in children undergoing operations.

RIGHT *Playing with other musicians is enjoyable and diverting.*

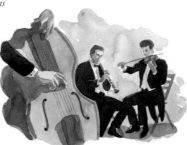

EFFECTIVENES

One study, using music therapy fo elderly depressed patients, reported that there was a greater improvement in symptoms in the group receiving music therapy tha in the control group.

SIDE-EFFECTS

None.

TREATMENT

Individual.

RELAXATION THERAPY

Learning a simple relaxation technique is a good way of helping to relieve stress and anxiety. Practicing it for only ten to twenty minutes a day is enough to be beneficial. The result is to slow breathing, reduce heart rate and lower muscle tension.

One approach to relaxation is to lie down on a mat on the floor, close your eyes and start to breathe slowly as if going to sleep. Let your arms fall out and away from your body with the palms facing upwards, and let your legs fall slightly apart. Tense and then relax each group of muscles for a few seconds in turn, perhaps starting at the feet, and working up the legs and trunk to the arms, neck and face. In this way, the whole body progressively becomes relaxed. Breathe in as you tense the muscles, then breathe out slowly and allow your muscles to relax. Imagine a pleasant, peaceful setting while you do this, such as lying on a sunny beach. As time goes on, it will be possible to learn to relax each muscle group in turn without first tensing them. Once the whole body is relaxed, spend about five or ten minutes in that state, breathing slowly and deeply.

BELOW *Relaxation techniques should be used every day to benefit.*

EFFECTIVENESS

Relieves stress and calms anxiety. Good in conjunction with other therapies.

SIDE-EFFECTS

None.

TREATMENT

Through visualization, deep breathing, tensing and relaxing of muscles. May also take the form of flotation therapy, where the client floats in a custom-built flotation tank of salty water, sometimes in complete darkness. Not suitable for claustrophobics.

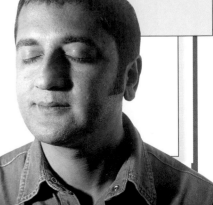

PRACTICAL TIPS FOR SUFFERERS

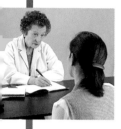

ABOVE *See your physician as a first step to treatment.*

It is vital that when you are unwell and experience persistent unpleasant symptoms, an orthodox medical practitioner is consulted. Certain rare physical causes of depression need to be excluded, for which there are specific treatments that will solve the problem and also remove the depression.

For example, a disorder of the endocrine system can produce depression as one of its effects. This can occur in people with an underactive thyroid gland.

Both cognitive behavior therapy and antidepressant drugs can treat depression effectively. Therefore, they should be taken seriously as an option. Various complementary therapies can indeed help. For St. John's wort, exercise, and to a lesser extent acupuncture and massage therapy, there is good evidence. Other complementary treatments may prove to be useful adjuncts to a conventional treatment plan.

LIFESTYLE

Often, interacting factors play a part in depression. Review lifestyle issues such as diet, exercise, alcohol consumption, activities, social life, and practical and emotional problems. This holistic approach looks at the whole person, rather than just concentrating on isolated symptoms.

THE WHOLE PICTURE

Good health can be seen as resulting from a positive interaction between mind, body, and surroundings. Emotional, practical, and biological aspects all need to be examined and dealt with. Health is not just the absence of disease, but may be described as a state of physical, emotional, and spiritual well-being.

Try and change bad lifestyle habits to those which enhance health. This process is not necessarily a particularly easy one, but the effort involved can be extremely worthwhile. It may be possible to get help from friends, relatives, orthodox and complementary health professionals, social services and self-help groups, to assist with a variety of problems ranging from housing difficulties to emotional problems. By looking at your lifestyle, you can take charge of aspects of your life, and enhance feelings of self-worth and well-being.

BELOW *Look at all the factors affecting you.*

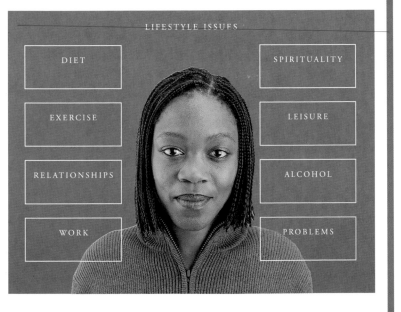

LIFESTYLE ISSUES

DIET

EXERCISE

RELATIONSHIPS

WORK

SPIRITUALITY

LEISURE

ALCOHOL

PROBLEMS

DAILY ACTIVITY

Exercise is linked to the improvement of the symptoms of mild to moderate depression, as well as having other health benefits. How much exercise are you taking? Do you spend most of the day sitting down, tend to use elevators instead of stairs, rarely walk anywhere, use the car or public transport most of the time, and take exercise less than three times a week? If so, it is likely that your health would benefit from more exercise. When you are depressed, it can be difficult to think things through clearly, make decisions, and to get started doing anything.

One advantage of physical activity is that it is not very demanding mentally. Once started, it provides a

BELOW *Remaining busy during the day helps to keep depression at bay.*

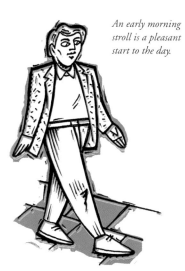

An early morning stroll is a pleasant start to the day.

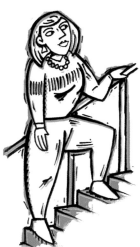

The routines of housework can be distracting.

distraction from worrying thoughts and is absorbing in itself. It's a good idea to start off gently with a pleasant activity such as gardening, walking, or cycling. You'll benefit from a sense of achievement when you've finished weeding a flower bed, or have made a short shopping trip. Set yourself a modest schedule of things to do each day, increasing it as you recover.

> *Any form of exercise can be helpful for improving depression, and it does not have to be particularly vigorous or strenuous. To get other types of health benefits, a little more exertion will be needed.*

Exercise boosts endorphines and maintains physical fitness.

Seeing the results of your gardening labors can be rewarding.

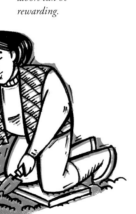

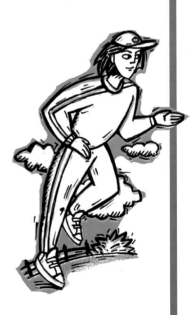

FOOD

The body needs a daily supply of food to provide the energy and nutrients necessary for it to maintain healthy tissues and organs, and to function properly. If you are severely depressed, you may lose your appetite and it can be a battle to eat at all, let alone to eat well. It is important to eat enough to keep the body going despite the effort required to prepare food.

Simple meals made from whole-wheat bread, fresh fruit and vegetables, and yogurt are wholesome and do not need much preparation. If it becomes too much to prepare meals, soluble nutritious powders for making into drinks (available at pharmacies) can be used as a temporary measure. Ideally a healthy diet is low in saturated fats and sugars, and high in fiber, fresh fruit and vegetables. A high saturated fat consumption is associated with heart and circulatory disease. However, although a healthy diet is something to aim for, the priority in depression is to continue to eat enough to maintain the body and provide adequate energy.

QUICK MEALS

When you are feeling at your worst, choose meals that are easily prepared, yet nutritious.

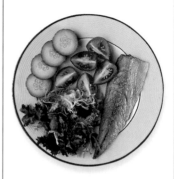

SIMPLE SALAD
Smoked mackerel, lollo rosso, tomatoes and cucumber slices.

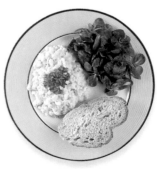

EASY EGGS
Scrambled eggs with parsley, salad greens, and wholewheat bread.

ALCOHOL

Alcohol acts as a depressant on the nervous system, any initial euphoria soon disappears, and there is a tendency to drink more to top up. Too much alcohol can produce anxiety and depression and may trigger aggression. Excess drinking is associated with a group of other health problems. Alcohol is also likely to cause problems if taken in conjunction with antidepressant drugs.

How do you know if you are drinking too much? If you answer yes to two or more of the following questions, then it is likely that your drinking is causing problems.

• *Have you ever thought that you should cut down on your drinking?*
• *Have you been annoyed by people criticizing your drinking?*
• *Have you ever felt guilty about your drinking?*
• *Have you ever taken a drink first thing in the morning to get rid of a hangover?*

ALCOHOL LIMITS

❖

Women should not drink more than fourteen units of alcohol a week.

❖

Men should not take more than twenty-one units a week.

❖

One unit consists of about a bottle of ordinary strength beer, or one glass of wine, or one measure of spirits. If you are depressed, it might be wise to reduce these general limits even further.

BELOW *Avoid the numbing temptations of alcohol: your problems will remain.*

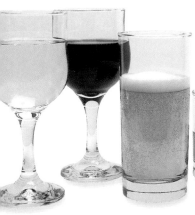

PRACTICAL TIPS FOR FAMILY AND FRIENDS

The experience of being depressed is a frightening and isolating one. It is hard to understand what it is like if you have not been through it yourself. At times, many depressed people want to talk about their feelings with someone they can trust.

HELP BY LISTENING

This can be painful for the listener, but it helps the depressed person to feel cared for and understood. In addition it provides an insight into depression for those who listen. Each sufferer's experiences are individual, but not everyone will want to talk about them. This must be respected. Friends and relatives should be sensitive to whether or not the sufferer wants to talk. It helps to spend more time listening, rather than talking and offering advice yourself.

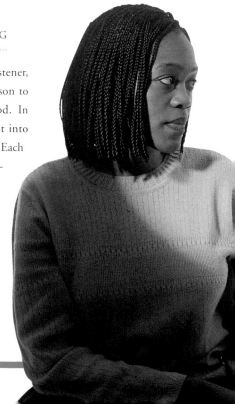

Being critical is unhelpful, as are well-meant comments such as "try to pull yourself together." People who are depressed have not chosen the experience, and they are not imagining their illness. If the depressed person talks about being suicidal it is important to take it seriously, and to seek professional help.

Providing support and sympathy can be draining, and it is necessary to keep up your own life and interests, and give yourself enough time for rest and relaxation. Local support groups for carers can be a useful way of discussing feelings and difficulties with others in the same situation.

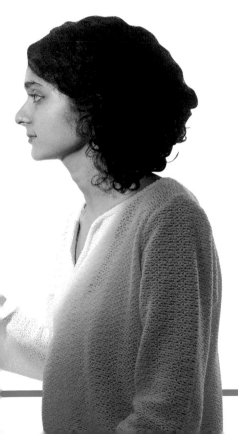

LEFT *Depressed people need their friends more than ever.*

PROFESSIONAL HELP

Encourage the depressed person to see his or her physician, as a first step.

Obtain a list of local reputable complementary therapists from the relevant professional bodies (look in the library), or ask your physician for suggestions.

Approach a local support group for help and advice.

Get professional help immediately if the sufferer talks of suicide.

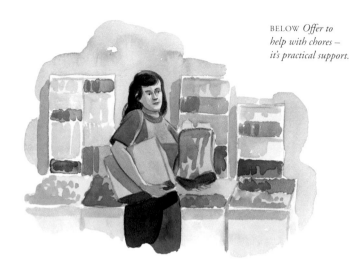

BELOW *Offer to help with chores – it's practical support.*

PROVIDE PRACTICAL SUPPORT

Energy, and the ability to concentrate, tend to be lower in depression. The sufferer can find it difficult to carry out everyday tasks. Offer to help with day-to-day chores: ask what would be most useful. Things such as helping with shopping, childcare or meal preparation can be very productive ways of giving assistance.

A depressed person may be difficult to support, and will often find it hard to ask for help. As the person recovers, it is important to let him gradually start doing things again for himself, so that self-confidence and independence are regained. You can help by supporting the sufferer in setting realistic goals to achieve, according to the severity of the depression. These goals should be reachable given the condition of the sufferer, or otherwise they can act to reinforce a sense of failure. It should be remembered that even a simple task, such as making a cup of coffee, can be a real achievement for someone floundering in the midst of depression.

PROVIDE EMOTIONAL SUPPORT

The existence of a supportive confiding relationship is beneficial to those suffering from depression. When depressed it can be hard to see any hope for the future, so reassurance that depression is only a temporary condition, that recovery will take place over time and things will improve, is important.

It can be difficult living with someone with depression as it is common for emotional withdrawal and inactivity to occur. The sufferer is no longer able to interact with others in the usual way, and it is easy for others to feel rejected. Depression is an illness where this withdrawal is characteristic, and it is not done deliberately to hurt people. Carers need patience and understanding to cope with this aspect. A carer's positive attitude and a gentle approach can promote the recovery process.

It can be difficult for the sufferer to be aware of improvements as they take place, so it can help if you notice and point out any positive changes along the road to recovery. Carers can provide a link to the outside world and so reduce feelings of isolation. They can help the sufferer to not completely lose touch with others. However, a depressed person tires easily and is likely to find it difficult to be with other people. What is helpful to one person may not be for another, but understanding, reassurance, a balanced diet, exercise, relaxation, and agreeable music are beneficial to most.

> ### HOW TO HELP
>
> ✧ Be patient.
> ✧ Be ready to listen when the sufferer wants to talk.
> ✧ Listen rather than offering advice.
> ✧ Don't be critical.
> ✧ Be supportive.
> ✧ Offer gentle sympathy.
> ✧ Volunteer to help with tasks.

LEFT *Encourage your friend to look ahead to a positive future.*

CHOOSING A COMPLEMENTARY THERAPIST

It is crucial to remember to consult your general physician before starting a new therapy and to keep in touch throughout it. Try to make sure that your expectations are realistic, and that you do not anticipate an instant cure.

ABOVE *Don't be over-optimistic when you go to a therapist.*

It is far more likely that the chosen complementary therapies might help to alleviate symptoms, or make it easier to live with the problem.

FINDING THE RIGHT THERAPIST FOR YOU

The therapist must not only be competent, but also someone who you are comfortable enough with to build up a good working relationship, as you will be seeing him or her regularly. It is important to check the credentials of the practitioner. This may not

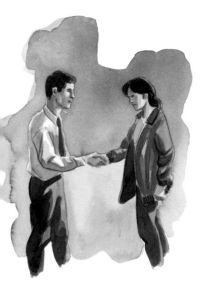

LEFT *You must feel comfortable with the therapist, if treatment is to be successful.*

always be straightforward, as many different certificates and qualifications exist. Check to see if the therapist belongs to an umbrella organization for the therapy. (But remember that membership may not guarantee quality and good practice. Find out a few facts about the professional body concerned. For instance, how does it assess the competence and the training undergone by its members? Does it have a code of ethics, complaints and disciplinary procedures, and a requirement for members to take out indemnity insurance?)

PRACTITIONER CHECKLIST

Before embarking on a course of therapy, ask the therapist some preliminary questions. Reputable therapists will be willing to discuss these basic issues at the outset. If not, it should set your alarm bells ringing.

What are your qualifications?
✧
How long have you practiced?
✧
Which professional body do you belong to?
✧
How useful do you think that the treatment is likely to be for depression?
✧
Of what exactly does the therapy consist?
✧
What side-effects may occur?
✧
How many sessions do you think may be necessary?
✧
Are you fully covered by insurance?
✧
How much will it cost?

ORTHODOX SOURCES OF HELP

When suffering from symptoms which might be depression, it is vital that the first port of call is your physician, so that a full assessment can be made. As already discussed, proven orthodox treatments exist for depression, including a variety of drugs and psychological treatment. If necessary, a general physician can refer you for a specialist opinion, and is also well placed to provide advice about other sources of help, both orthodox and voluntary. However, the amount of knowledge about, and attitude to, complementary therapies varies greatly among individual physicians.

Other orthodox sources of help include the community mental health team, clinical psychologists, counselors and social workers. Community psychiatric nurses can give support and advice, and make home visits. Social workers may be able to help with housing, financial, and employment difficulties. A counselor is available at some physicians' practices. Self-help groups may exist in your area for those who suffer or have suffered from depression, or for families and carers. Information about these should be available from your physician, the local library, or direct from national organizations.

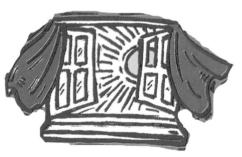

HELPFUL BOOKS

Butler, B., and Hope, A.
*Manage Your Mind. The Mental
Health Fitness Guide.*
(Oxford University Press, UK, 1995.)

Copeland, M.A.
*Living Without Depression And
Manic Depression.*
(New Harbinger Publications,
US, 1995.)

Madders, J.
Stress And Relaxation.
(Macdonald Optima, UK, 1981.)

McCormick, E.W.
*Coping, Healing And Rebuilding After
Nervous Breakdown.*
(Optima, UK, 1993.)

Payne, R.A.
Relaxation Techniques.
(Churchill Livingstone, UK, 1995.)

Rosenthal, N.E.
Winter Blues.
(Guildford Press, UK, 1994.)

Rowe, D.
*Depression: The Way
Out Of Your Prison.*
(Routledge, UK, 1996.)

Smith, G., and Nairne, K.
Dealing With Depression.
(The Women's Press, UK, 1995.)

Rowlands, B.
*The Which? Guide To
Complementary Medicine.*
(Which? Books, UK, 1997.)

Sanders, P., and Myers, S.
*What Do You Know About Depression
And Mental Health?*
(Gloucester Press, UK, 1996.)
Aimed at young
people.